DUAL DIAGNOSIS

HOW TO OVERCOME THE CHALLENGES OF DUAL DIAGNOSIS

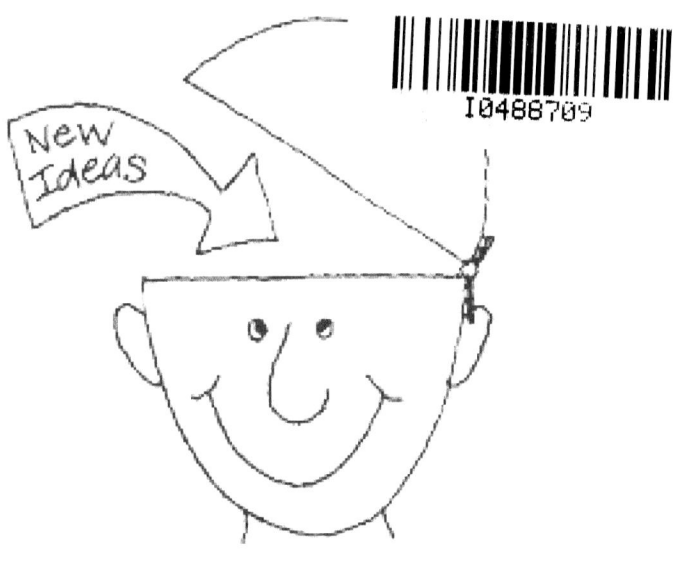

By Patricia A Carlisle

Introduction

I want to thank you and congratulate you for choosing the book, *"**DUAL DIAGNOSIS: How to overcome the challenges of Dual Diagnosis**"*.

Dual diagnosis is a common phenomenon affecting the modern day societies of the world. What is really responsible for the syndrome? There are a few reasons why many societies are witnessing the problem. But what is the meaning of dual diagnosis? How do we deal with the challenges associated with dual diagnosis? To start with, Dual diagnosis can be referred to as that condition that brings about the simultaneous existence, and mental illness at the same time, a problem which assumes a dual nature. This condition appears to look like something that can further lead to more heterogeneous problem.

However, the issue has led to many debates whether it is possible for someone to suffer similar faith of dual problems, and yet still be referred to as a single problem. Experience has however, shown that it is very possible for an individual to suffer problems that assume a dual nature other than a single problem.

In the distant example we have problems associated with dual diagnosis to be seen to manifest in critical conditions like alcoholism and depression. This is a very good example of a problem that has to do with dual diagnosis. The condition can also be seen in a more serious mental illness like schizophrenia and psychosis. It can also manifest in conditions that has to do with substance misuse when it leads to development of certain disorders too, for instance, when an individual over use cannabis.

Other forms of disorders that can lead to dual diagnosis problems are panic disorders, generalized anxiety disorders, and over dependence on drugs. It is however to be noted that substance abuse can on its own lead to a problem which can be regarded as self induced, and it exist separately from a pre-existing mental illness or psychiatric.

Persons with dual diagnosis problems always face complexities of problems such as, a high rate of relapse, frequent hospitalization is a common phenomenon for some parts of the world, it can further lead to homelessness, and can even further worsen to non-conforming societal behavior which is abhorred in contacting dreadful diseases such as, HIV/ AIDS, Hepatitis, and other sexually transmittable diseases. The causes of co-occurring disorders are yet to be fully determined, but there are several propositions and theories that have been put forward by experts in the field of diagnosis.

Thanks again for choosing this book, I hope you enjoy it!

ABOUT THE AUTHOR

Patricia A. Carlisle, MSW, CBT

Patricia Carlisle- a Master in Social Work and Cognitive Behavioral Therapist (CBT) gives out an expression of how important it is for an individual to take into consideration the concept of self-assessment to know what human, technical and conceptual skills they posses to perform or to achieve what they desire, or to deal with everyday life. However, every particular group of people has their own unique set of ideas, traditions and events including the frame of mind according to which people perform but there are many who faces problems and fail to maintain a healthy mind set affecting their behaviors and performance to those around them.

People like Patricia Carlisle are among those who have felt this urge of serving people and helping them out of their mental crisis towards a healthy life. She has experienced some close encounters in her personal life regarding mental health issues in her family and friends that has encouraged her to pursue this as her career.

Currently Patricia Carlisle is serving as a Certified On-Line Cognitive Behavioral Therapist with an extensive 15years of experience using Cognitive-Behavior Therapy Techniques. She envisions a world where everyone gets mental health treatment with no mental health stigma and to make it real she has already set up her own Holistic Measure Online Comprehensive Behavioral Healthcare Company after retiring from The Nord Center in The Partial Hospitalization Program (PHP) Dept for 5 years and Murtis H. Taylor Mental Health Center as a mental health counselor, psychological support technician and case manager for 10 years to emulsify her skills more professionally.

Along with this, she has wrote down her passion as a clinician in 25 or more short books to help individuals and families get their life back, freeing them of the restraints of negative thinking, anxiety and depression by using different approaches. She is highly appreciated among her clients for her flexibility and professionalism of dealing with them graciously. To reach her, make use of her direct website address: http://therapist2013.wix.com/e-therapy . As she is ready to inspire hope and contribute to health and well-being by providing the best online health care through comprehensive practice, education and research.

TABLE OF CONTENT

Chapter 1

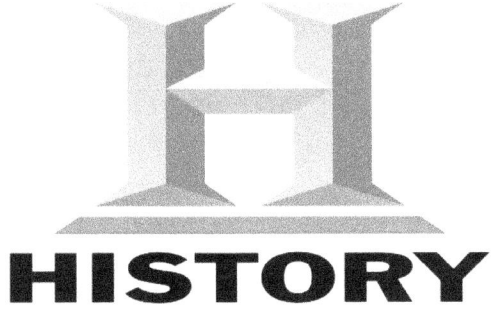

HISTORY

HISTORICAL BACKGROUND

The original approach for treating persons with the problem, or suffering from dual diagnosis was a comparable treatment program which was very popular, and which method was adapted as the right approach. In this system, the patients received mental health provisions which started from one clinician; meanwhile, the addressing of the substance abuse was done with a different medical professional.

Researchers have since discovered that the comparable treatment were not effective, but they made references to the need to join, or integrate the services of treating mental health with issues concerning substance abuse, and also address the issue systematically. In the mid 1980s, some of the propositions began to join substance abuse services and mental health services in a offer to meet the demands and needs of the day.

The system worked to move the treatment approach for substance abuse from an offensive approach to a much more supportive approach. New methods and innovation were also adopted which includes motivating clients or patients, and working with them to form a long term aims and goals which will further assist in taking care of them effectively.

However, the research studies carried out of the said initiatives did not take care of possess control groups, the results obtained were however promising which then become the basis, or bedrock for emergent efforts aimed at developing and studying more approaches and methods for bringing more integrated treatment approaches to health practitioners.

Chapter 2

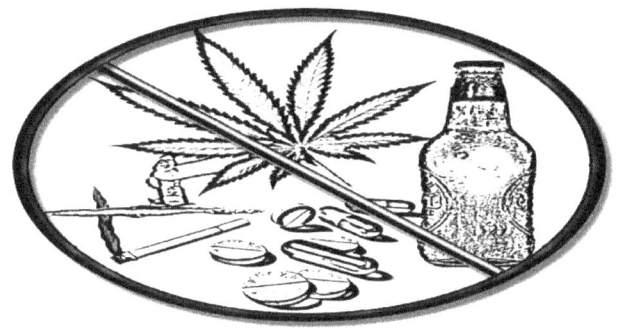

PRE-EXISTING DIAGNOSIS AND SUBSTANCE INDUCE DIAGNOSIS

Symptomatology which is caused by the effects of excessive drug abuse, and can also includes alcohol abuse that tends to resembles mental illness, but actually is not, seem to create confusion. It is self induced, and is different from a pre-existing condition of mental illness, and sometimes when that dual nature exist before treatment it tends to create a lot of problem during the treatment. When there is a prolong abstinence from alcohol and drugs, there is the tendency that the psychiatric disorders begins to reduce, and disappear when there is a measure of control or withdrawal from the intake of alcohol and drugs.

Therefore, substance abuse disorders leads to mood changes and distortion that are generally referred to as substance-induced mood disorders. There are also other disorders that are induced by other substance that lead to, or causes anxiety disorders and the overlapping or existence of this kind, or problems normally leads to the existence or effects of a dual diagnosis problem.

Chapter 3

HOW TO TREAT DUAL DIAGNOSIS

Some people who have co-occurring disorders do receive enough treatment for dual diagnosis problem. It was evaluated in year 2011 that only about 12.4 per cent of American matured individuals with the problem of co-occurring disorders had received subsequent mental health and addiction treatment. Patients with dual diagnosis disorders were experiencing difficult challenges in getting access to treatment and facilities, quite often, they have been excluded from mental health facilities, whenever they admit to having problems with substance abuse, and so on and so forth.

There are several methods to treat concurrent disorders which fit the subject matter of this book. Initially, treating the problem partially involves treating the disorders that can be said to be the primary disorder. Subsequently, after the treatment of the primary disordered (i.e. one of the co-occurring disorder) then follows the treating of the secondary disorder, but this will be done after the stabilization of the primary disorder. Other similar treatment involves the patient receiving mental health consultancy services or treatment from an expert, while the addictions treatment should be handled by another expert different from the initial expert, or separate from the one treating the primary co-occurring disorder.

Joining the treatment involves making use of a systematic blending of series of interventions into a particular or specific coherent. And, careful treatment developed with regular ideology and systematic approach or method among health providers. This method will help us to see that both disorders are primary in nature. So, joining treatment can lead to an improvement in accessibility, service personification, engaging in treatment, symptoms of mental health, compliance treatment method, and above all outcomes that will be analyzed positively.

Organizations like the **"SUBSTANCE ABUSE AND MENTAL HEALTH SERVICES ADMINISTRATION"**, based in the U.S., described joining or integrating treatment is in the very best interest of both patient, funders, programs, and the entire system that is used in the operation. It was further propose that the treatments and collaboration processes between the patients and the team of health services providers should work with mutual understanding and care. Moreover, recovery process should be perceived as a long race rather than a short walk, and the approaches and results, or aims and goals should be clear and well spelt out by the institution or organization that is running the operation whether it is governmental, or non-governmental organization.

.

Chapter 4

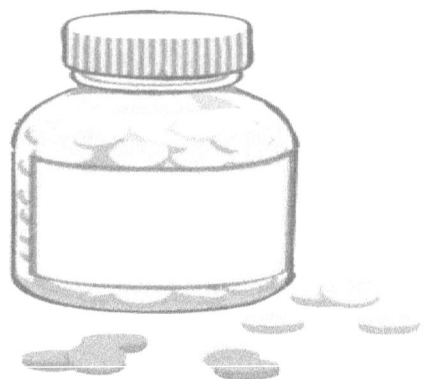

MEDICATION APPROACH

Sometimes, a lot of patients do not accept medication as antithetical to substance abuse rehabilitation, and the adverse effects, although they can be very good to reduce anxiety, paranoia and craving. Scientific medications that have positively worked effectively include opioid substation therapies, like lifelong preservation, maintenance, buprenorphine, or methadone, to reduce the adverse effects of relapse, critical and legitimate trouble involving opioid addicted individuals as well as assisting them with cravings.

Alcohol addicts, cocaine addicts, opioid addicts, and amphetamine addicts have baclofen which will also help them to eliminate the cravings for drugs. These are the approaches to the treatments. Other approaches include the use of Clozapine which is antipsychotic; this is used in minimizing the use of illegal drug that has been ingested by patients into their body system as a stimulant. Clozapine is responsible for some traces of respiratory problem when it is used in combination with alcohol, so it is being discouraged to use Clozapine. Hence, try as much as possible to avoid Clozapine for treatment of dual diagnosis problem. And it is always advisable to always consult expert advice for a successful handling of any critical case.

Chapter 5

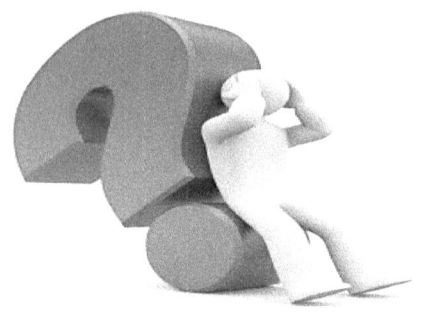

DUAL DIAGNOSIS THEORIES

Several theories trying to explain and determine the relationship between substance abuse and mental abuse resulting in the dual diagnosis problem today. We shall have a look at the following Theory as put forward.

The Casualty Theory

This theory proposes that there are certain kinds of substance abuse that may temporarily, or casually cause mental illness. There are persuasive evidence that using cannabis is capable of temporarily causing psychotic effect, and experiences on the mentality of users. If this is persistent, there is usually a continuous effect; there is always an increase in the problem of psychotic outcomes in affected people involved in cannabis ingestion. This theory is still being study over the last couple of years.

There are other theories like the super-sensitivity theory; Autism spectrum disorder, Attention-deficit hyperactivity disorder, past exposure to psychiatric medications theory; Self-medication theory, Alleviation of dysphoria theory, and multiple risk factor theory have also been put forward by practitioners.

Chapter 6

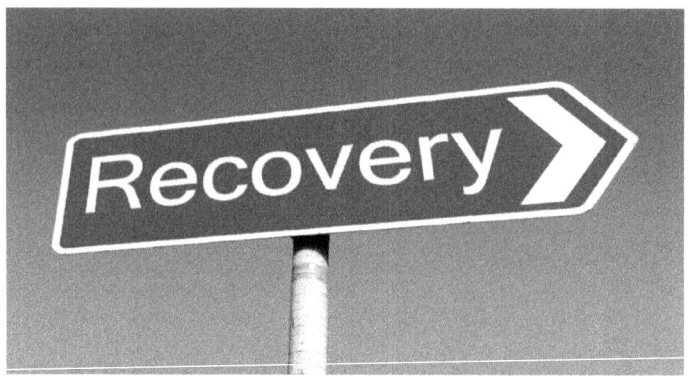

OVERCOMING DUAL DIAGNOSIS

As earlier discussed, dual diagnosis problem is very difficult to handle sometimes. The problem is better handle by not just one expert, but two or more experts who are skilled, and are in a better position to handle the case. Treating dual diagnosis as an expert involved taking several approaches as we have discussed earlier. But if the case is handled by a professional, it is expected that the procedures will be taken in order to achieve success must be followed to the later.

The first method is arresting and isolating the primary source, or first co-occurring disorder, treating it first, then when that aspect has been successfully dealt with, the secondary co-occurring disorder can be gradually treated accordingly. The experts are always expected to be in charge of any situation, and should always make sure that they deliver the best practices. Funding for such dual diagnoses is always viewed as something that is very costly, and most government are always of the opinion that despite the fact that they have huge responsibilities of delivering quality health care to the people, they also deserve to work within the available budget that will help in maximizing efficiency of resources.

Persons with mental illnesses are recognized by law, and that is why we have the psychiatric hospitals being managed and operated by the Government. The treatment for such people under mental health care are always given consideration above other kinds of psychotic problems derived from substance ingestion, such as hard drugs like cocaine, cannabis, opium etc. individuals affected by hard drugs and alcoholism problems are always viewed as persons who are irresponsible. How many of those irresponsible people who have inflicted themselves with hard drugs and alcohol will the government be ready to take care of? That is one of the reasons that government will always admonished and give warning like; "drink responsibly," "don't drink and drive", and "tobacco smokers are liable to die young." Overcoming and coping with the challenges of dual diagnosis by health practitioners is very difficult, especially when the condition of the patient is critical, and has a chronic type of mental illness accompanied by substance abuse.

It is a pre-requisite requirement that health practitioners should always show empathy with clients. No matter how difficult the situation appears to be, it is best that we put into consideration the situation of the client, and we need to show a lot of care. Addiction caused by ingestion is always seen by people as something that is negative, and many occasion have proven that people do not like associating, or having anything to do with people with such problems.

Chapter 7

Biggest Challenge

OVERCOMING CHALLENGES OF DUAL DIAGNOSIS BY VICTIMS
Rehabilitation

While patients constitute the bulk of those who are suffering the syndrome, it is understandable that while they suffer the consequences of the primary aspect of the co-occurring disorders, if it is as a result of substance abuse or alcoholism, submitting once self to rehabilitation is the right step in the right direction. Rehabilitation is one of the keys to overcoming the challenge of dual diagnosis.

When a person has already become a victim, and it is noticeable that the health problem is there, it has been established that it has become a serious problem. The adverse health conditions can further lead to serious complications which can be detrimental to the health and life of the individual, so the best bet is to submit his or herself to medical rehabilitation treatment where the problem will be diagnosed and treated by experts who have the technical know how to handle the situation.

Expert Treatment

Persons suffering from dual disorders should seek expert advice for the right direction. It is usually recommended that health workers involved in the provisions of such services are to be given necessary details on the symptoms, and the patient should open up for the experts to be able to assist him or her to solve the problem whenever it arises. The time the problem began should be known as well as other disturbance the patient is going through should be explained to the expert to help them provide the right approach of treatment expected.

Positive Thinking

There is no miracle like personal conviction with the power of positive thinking. You need a strong faith and believe in yourself that the problem can be overcome with just a little effort. You need to have at the back of your mind that everything should be taken one step at a time, slow and steady wins the race, in other words, there is a need for the person to be patient with himself, there is no need to be hard on once self if you find yourself in such condition. All you need to do is believe that you will overcome the problem; that is the mindset and character that should be shown every time you face such challenges.

Stay away from Drugs

There is the need for you to avoid taking hard drugs that may further aggravate your efforts to get yourself back together again. You have to see the substance as your enemy, having at the back of our mind that the only reason why you are where you are, and facing the problem you are facing is the result of that cannabis or cocaine that you have been ingesting into your system.

Support You Mental Development

Education is one thing that can assist you in developing mentally, and it is very important to involved yourself in things that can edify the mind, you can chose to read books such as inspirational books, novels, and you can also join social media and forums to engage in discussions that will assist you to develop positively.

Secondly, join sporting groups and running groups, or visit the gym regularly to try to develop your mind both physically and mentally. Exercise is one important thing that will always assist you to develop your entire well being when it comes to physical education, we can go for this form of activities to further strengthen our resilience over substance abuse inclination. Activities as mentioned here is very good to help keep persons who are having challenges of dual diagnosis, and for those who are not having the problem, they can also avoid it by engaging in these activities which will further strengthen them to live a healthy lifestyle, and avoid a dual disorder.

Get involved in Family and Career

For some person who like leaving their family to join friends that can likely have a bad influence over them can further lead to destroying their lives. It is better to spend more time with your family than some gang, or group with questionable characters that will not help you in developing mentally or health-wise. But rather, spend more time with your family; having a united family forming one bond will further foster a better understanding.

Your career is also very important, you will not want to jeopardize your career with excessive drinking of alcohol causing you more depression, or taking hard drugs that can ruin your career. Many have been brought down from the mountain of success as a result of a boring attitude, and handling their career with kid gloves. This has led to further destruction and depreciation to their career and family life.

Conclusion

Thank you again for choosing this book!

I hope this book was able to help you to understand the importance of treating or caring for someone with duel diagnosis.

To overcome the challenges of dual diagnosis it takes a team of professionals because of the huge challenges involved in the processes in handling the situation. For instance, the government has a huge role to play by providing adequate well trained health workers and medical personnel to handle the situations, and also provide adequate health facilities, and working environment to help implementation and monitoring of the running of hospitals, and rehabilitation centers. Doctors have a lot to do in order to ensure that patients are treated and that the health conditions are always improving for the best.

Family members also have a role to play by supporting, and helping any of its members who has been experiencing the problem, schools and educational institutions cannot afford to seat back and watch the lives of their student destroyed by drug dealers. Hence, the need to offer adequate solution to the most important issues involved in the treatment involving dual diagnosis.

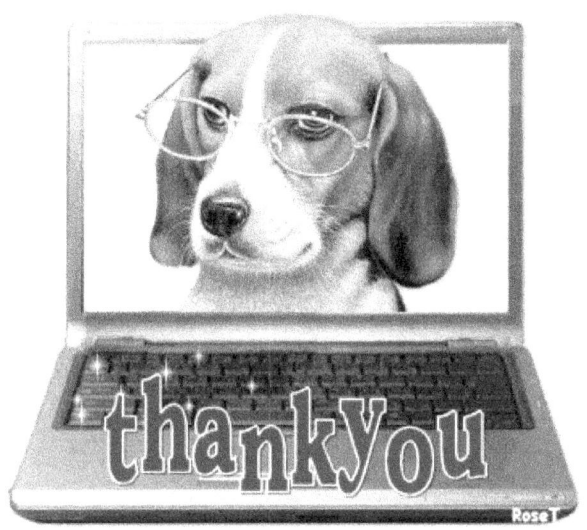

Finally, if you enjoyed this book, would you be kind enough to leave a review for this book on Amazon? It'd be greatly appreciated!

Thank you and good luck!

Preview Of 'THOUGHTS WITHOUT THINKING: Taking control over your racing thoughts'

Chapter 1: RACING THOUGHTS

Racing thoughts can be a problem. It's not simply the substance of the thoughts it's the way it feels. For example, your thoughts are moving at such a quick pace, and you can't remember what the last thought was, and yet another thought instantly takes its over. Racing thoughts can influence anyone with anxiety; however it is most commonly experienced in people that have anxiety attacks.

It's also extremely common at night before you go to sleep. For reasons unknown, numerous individuals discover their thoughts appear to race quicker when they're attempting to sleep. The reasons for racing thoughts are likely identified with the way your neurotransmitters interface aid your anxiety, couple with the surge of adrenaline you get when you have anxiety (which may make your mind significantly more active). Adrenaline, particularly, causes your psyche to be over-active while at the same time making it harder to center interest. Different reasons may include:

1) There are no distractions. When you're left with your own thoughts, your thoughts frequently go free, and in the end they are untamed.

2) Anxiety might also bring hyperventilation, which can incidentally bring less blood to the cerebrum. This is particularly common when experiencing an anxiety attack. It's likely that your mind is really not working, and you're having difficulty stopping the thoughts. Try not to stress-this isn't risky.

3) Lack of sleep is the main reason behind this. Anxiety can also stop you from sleeping, and the lack of sleep may also prompt racing thoughts. This can often become a self-satisfying issue, since anxiety prompts absence of rest which prompts racing thoughts which prompts an absence of rest. That is why most people seem to experience repeated thoughts and it becomes extremely upsetting.

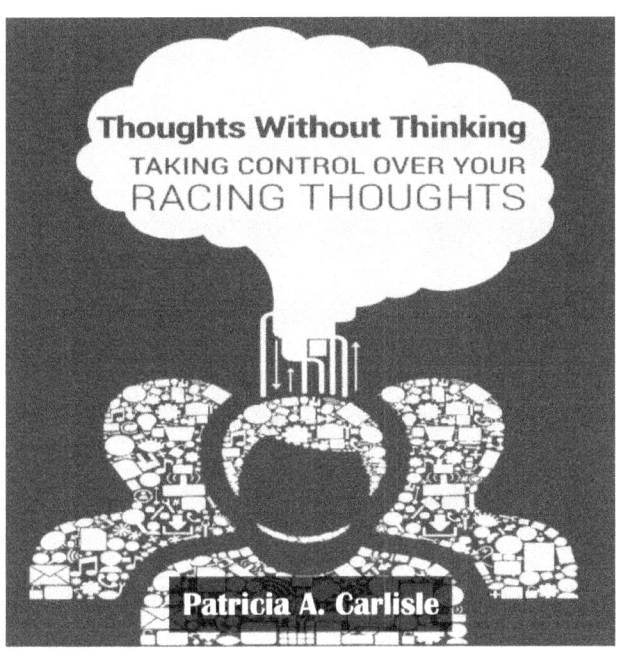

To read more about "THOUGHTS WITHOUT THINKING: Taking Control over Your Racing Thoughts. Go to Amazon.com

Check Out My Other Books

Below you'll find some of my other popular books that are popular on Amazon and Kindle as well. Alternatively, you can visit my author page on Amazon to see other work done by me.

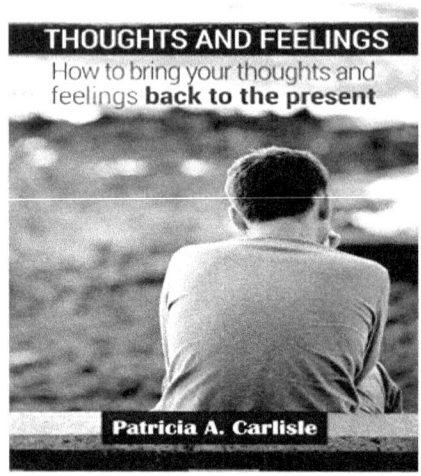

THOUGHTS AND FEELINGS: Hot to bring your thoughts and feelings back to the present.

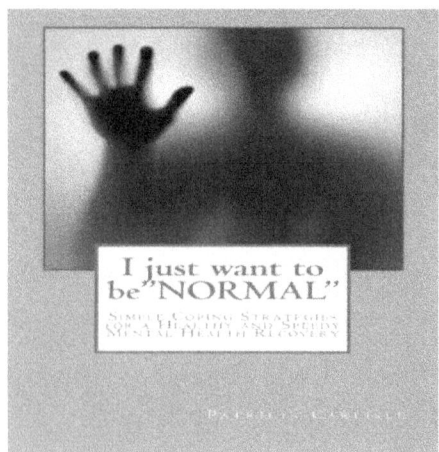

I just want to be "NORMAL." Simple Coping Strategies for a Healthy and Speedy Mental Health Recovery.

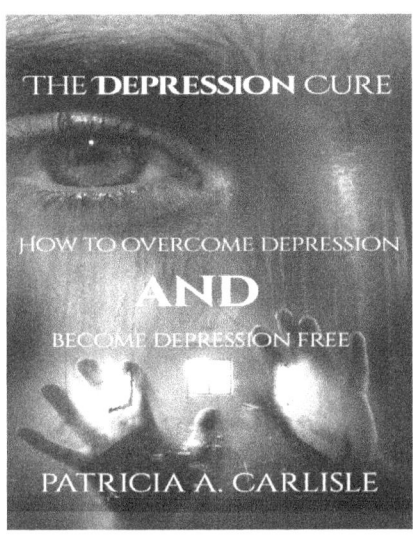

THE DEPRESSION CURE: How to Overcome Depression and Become Depression Free.

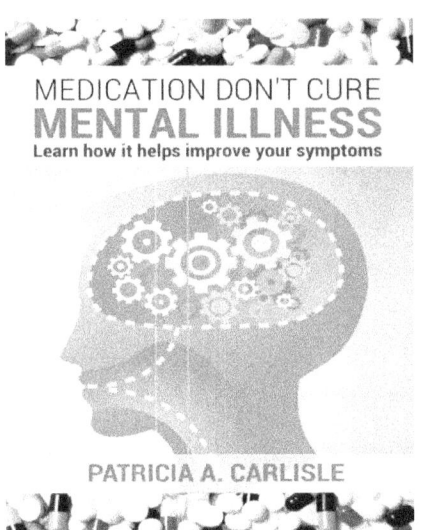

MEDICATION DON'T CURE MENTAL ILLNESS: Learn how it helps improve your symptoms.

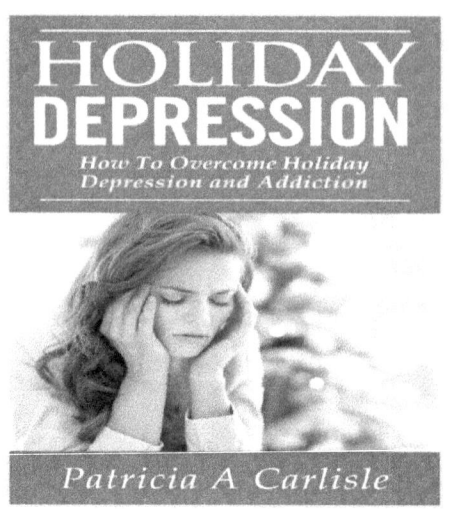

**HOLIDAY DEPRESSION: How To Overcome Holiday
Depression and Addiction.**

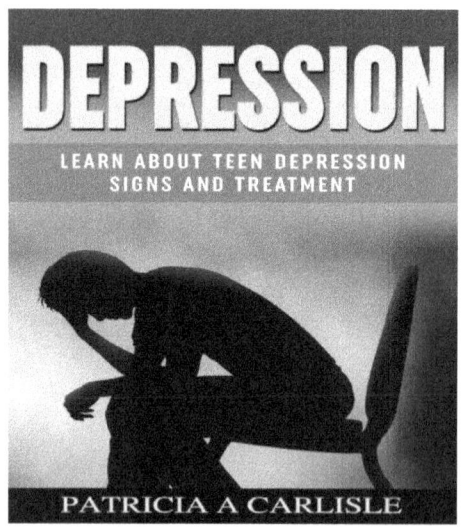

**DEPRESSION: Learn about teen depression signs
and treatment.**

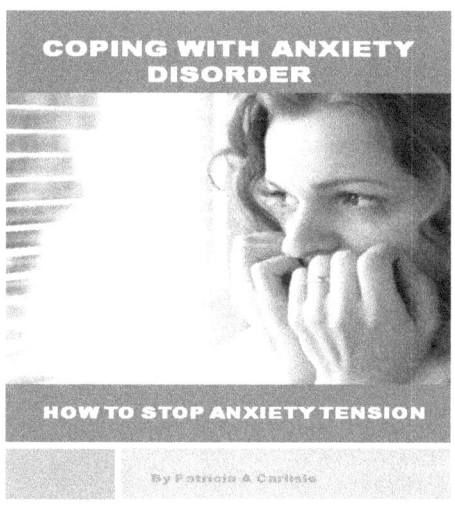

COPING WITH ANXIETY DISORDER: How to stop Anxiety Tension.

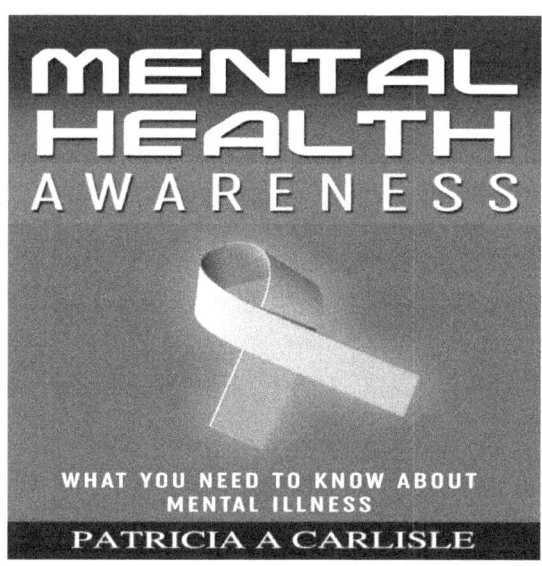

MENTAL HEALTH AWARENESS: WHAT YOU NEED TO KNOW ABOUT MENTAL ILLNESS.

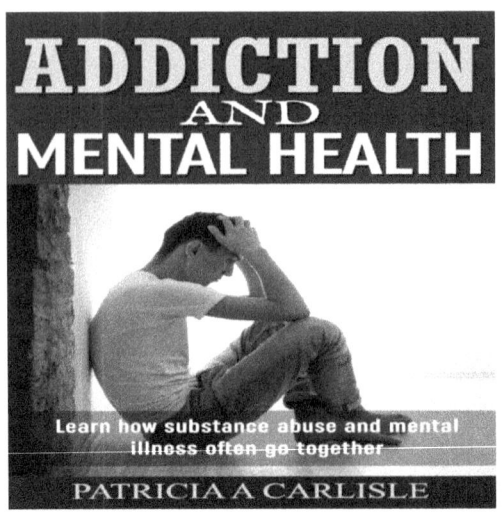

ADDICTION AND MENTAL HEALTH: Learn how substance abuse and mental illness often go together.

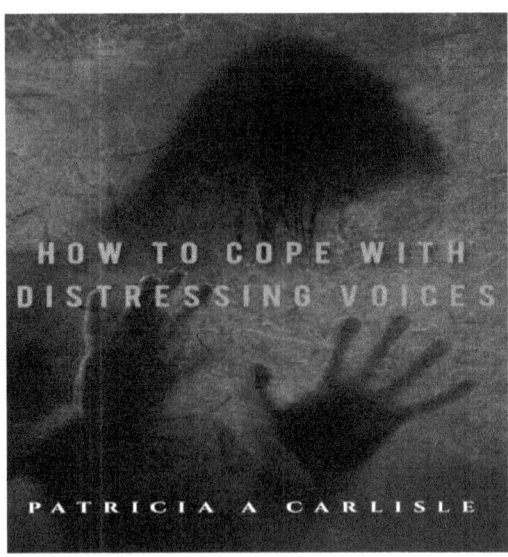

HOW TO COPE WITH DISTRESSING VOICES.

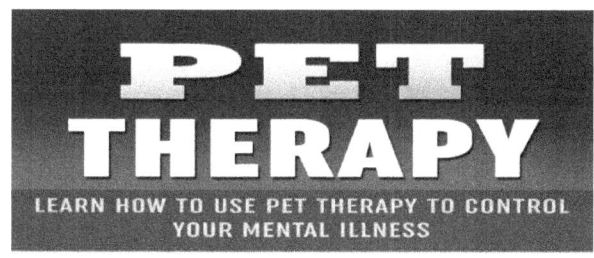

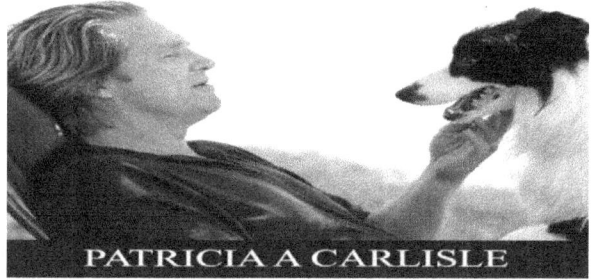

PET THERAPY: Learn How To Use Pet Therapy To Control Your Mental Illness.

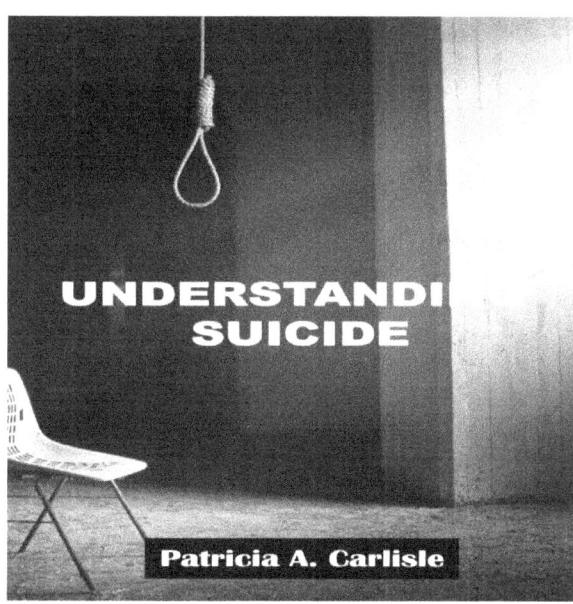

UNDERSTANDING SUICIDE.

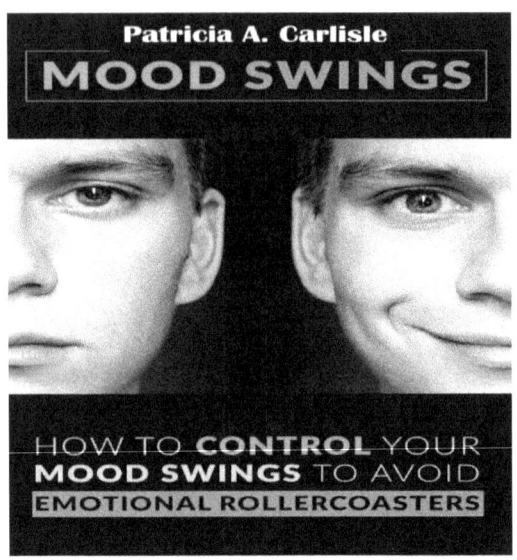

MOOD SWINGS: How to Control Your Mood Swings To Avoid Emotional Rollercoaster's.

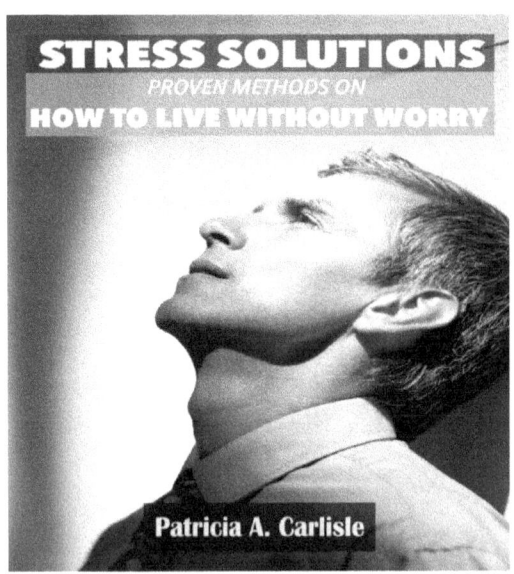

STRESS SOLUTIONS: Proven Methods On How To Live Without Worry.

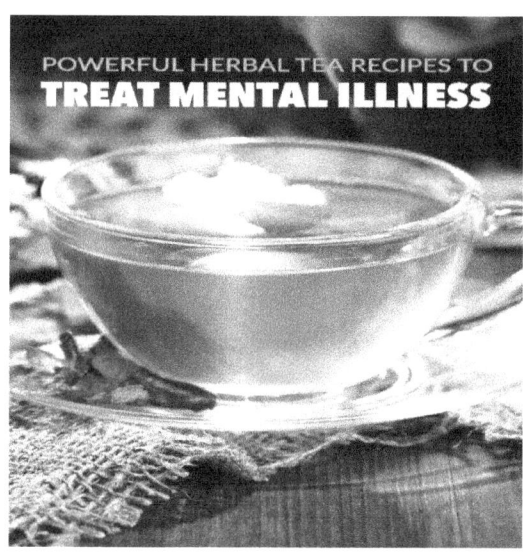

POWERFUL HERBAL TEA RECIPES TO TREAT MENTAL ILLNESS.

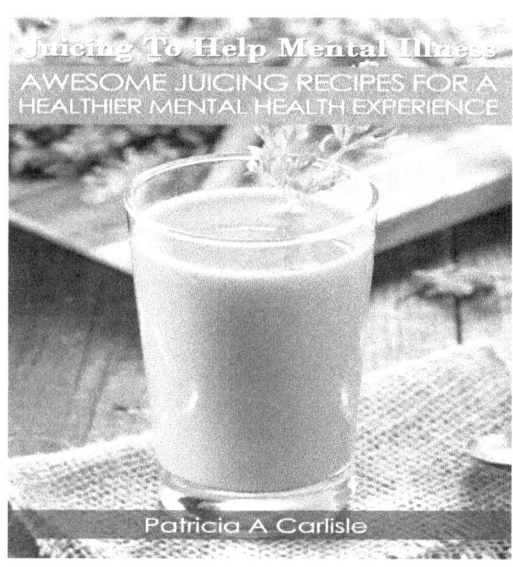

JUICING TO HELP MENTAL ILLNESS: Awesome Juicing Recipes For A Healthier Mental health Experience.

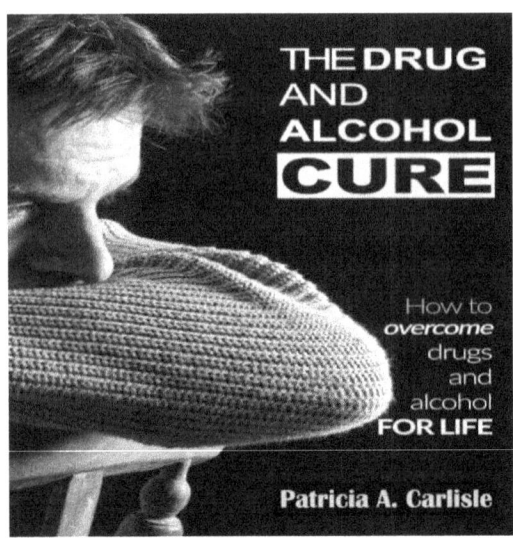

THE DRUG AND ALCOHOL CURE: How to Overcome Drugs and Alcohol for Life.

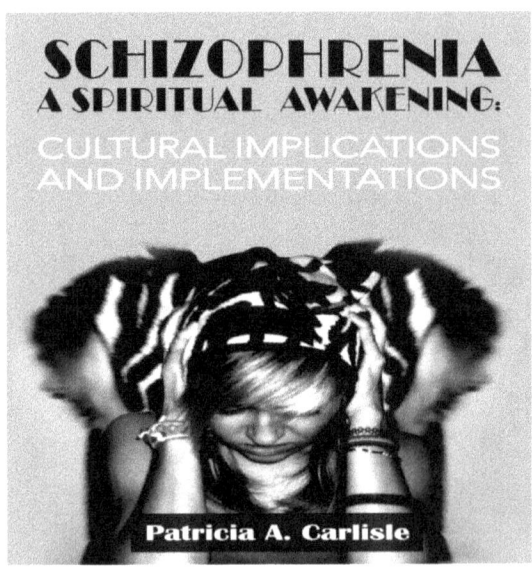

SCHIZOPHRENIA A SPIRITUAL AWAKENING: CULTURAL IMPLICATIONS AND IMPLEMENTATIONS.

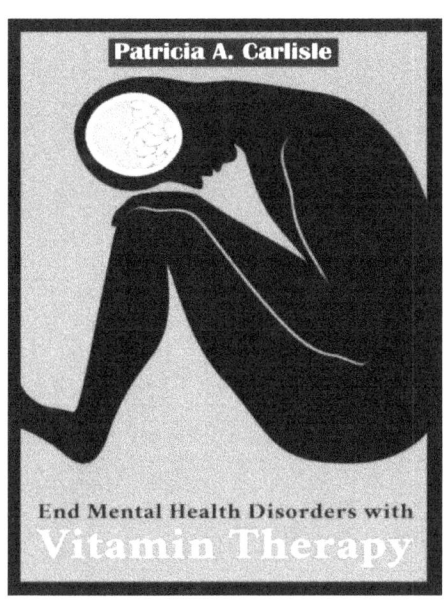

VITAMIN THERAPY: End Mental Health Disorders With vitamin Therapy.

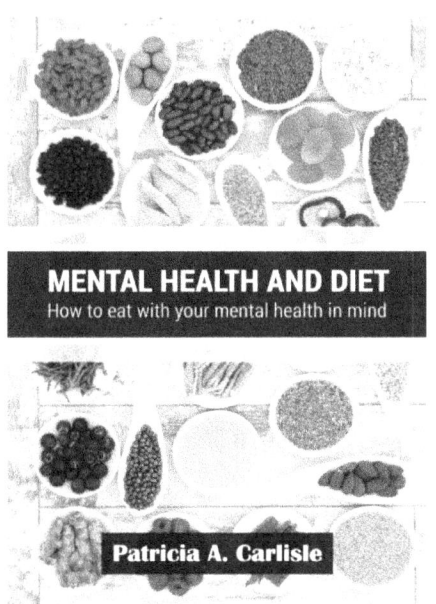

MENTAL HEALTH AND DIET: How to Eat With Your Mental Health In Mind.

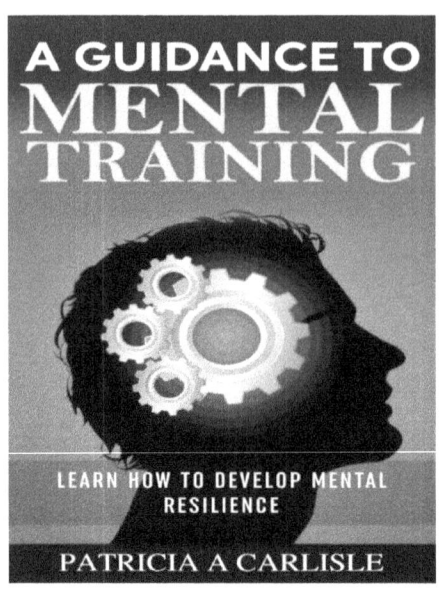

A GUIDANCE TO MENTAL TRAINING: Learn How To Develop Mental Resilience.

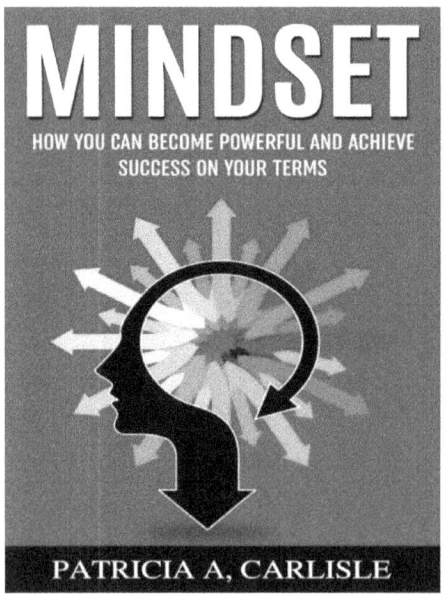

MINDSET: How You Can Become Powerful And Achieve success On Your Terms.

BONUS: SUBSCRIBE TO THE FREE BOOK

Beginners Guide to Yoga & Meditation

"Stressed out? Do You Feel Like The World Is Crashing Down Around You? Want To Take A Vacation That Will Relax Your Mind, Body And Spirit? Well this Easy To Read Step By Step

E-Book Makes It All Possible!"

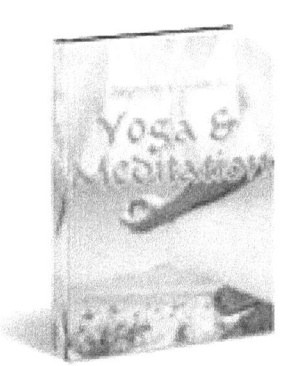

Instructions on how to join our mailing list, and receive a free copy of "Yoga and Meditation" can be found in any of my Kindle eBooks.

NOTES

NOTES

NOTES

NOTES

NOTES

NOTES

www.ingramcontent.com/pod-product-compliance
Lightning Source LLC
Chambersburg PA
CBHW071544170526
45166CB00004B/1552